January 27, 2019.
Thank you for your
support. God bless you!

Much love

Maxine A. Wilson

Zariah

Zariah's New Heart

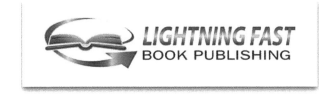

www.lfbookpublishing.com

Summary: A book which chronicles a young girl's journey of struggle and triumph in dealing with her heart ailment.

ISBN 10: 0-9994653-6-8
ISBN 13: 978-0-9994653-6-3

References
The International 22q11.2 Deletion Syndrome Foundation, Inc. website. Retrieved June 1,2005, www.22q.org

<u>Acknowledgement</u>

First, I would like to thank the Lord for laying upon my heart the need to write this book.

My thanks to family and friends for their support.

Officers Roger and Karen Hasty and Stephan and Ashlee Wildish of The Salvation Army for their Love, Support and Prayers during Zariah's heart operation.

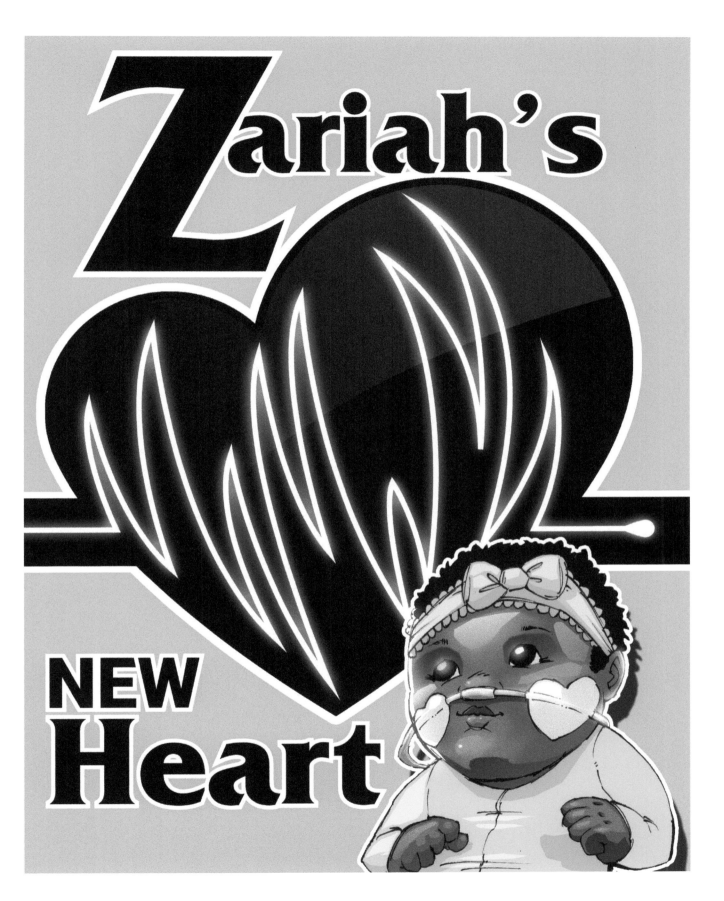

Zariah's NEW Heart

Written by Maxine A. Wilson, RN
Illustrated by Brian Gabourel

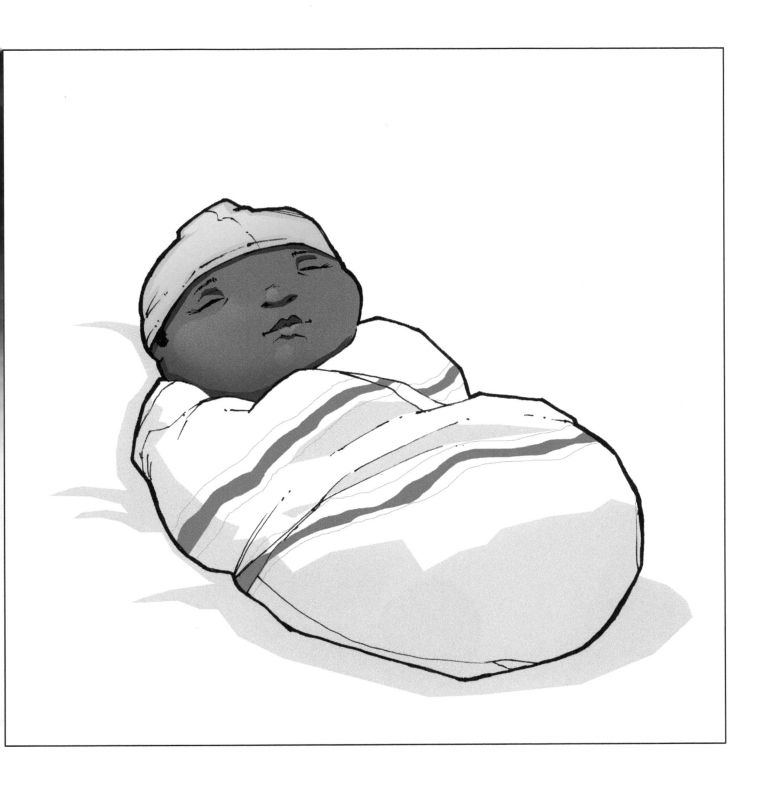

June 16, 2010

I am Zariah Wilson. I was born today at 08:01 PM on my great- grandfather's 81st birthday at
Prince George's Hospital. My mother was so happy to finally see me face to face after
39 weeks inside of her.

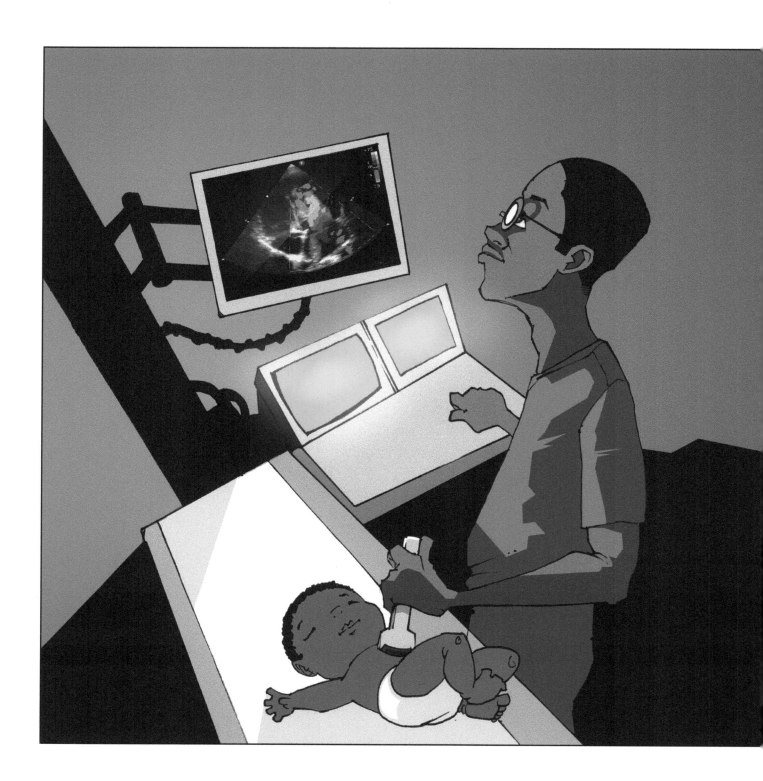

June 17, 2010

Dr. Wossen and the doctors at Children's National Medical Center took a picture of my heart; it's called an echocardiogram. They discovered that I have a condition called Tetralogy of Fallot, (TOF). It means I have a hole in my heart and extra tissue in the artery that goes to my lungs. My brain and body need oxygen. If enough blood does not go to my lungs to pick up oxygen and take it to the rest of my body, I could have Tet spells. During a Tet spell, I turn blue.

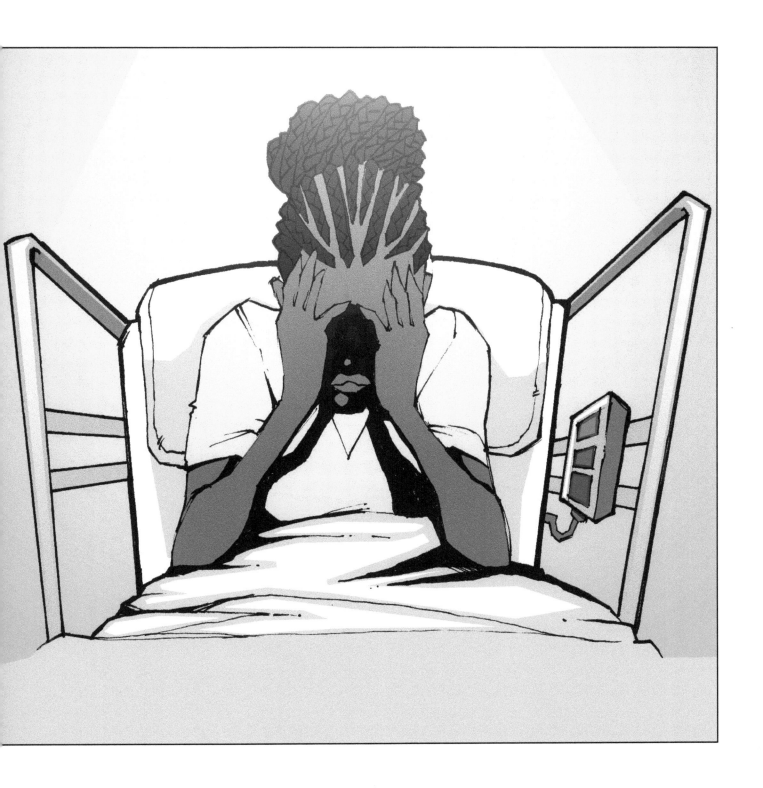

My mother was very sad, because I could not stay in her hospital room with her. I was placed in the nursery to have my oxygen level monitored with a pulse ox apparatus on my foot.

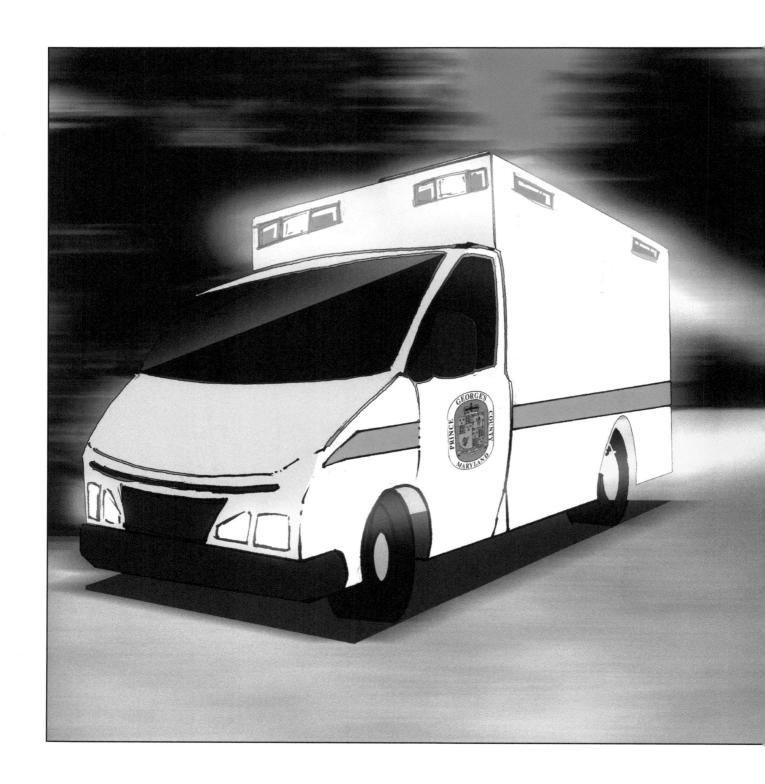

June 18, 2010

My First Ambulance Ride

Instead of going home, I was taken in an ambulance with my mother to Children's National Medical Center Heart and Kidney Unit to be monitored further. The nurses and doctors placed me on a monitor that recorded my heart rate, oxygen level, blood pressure and my respiratory rate. I was monitored for 3 days and then I was sent home.

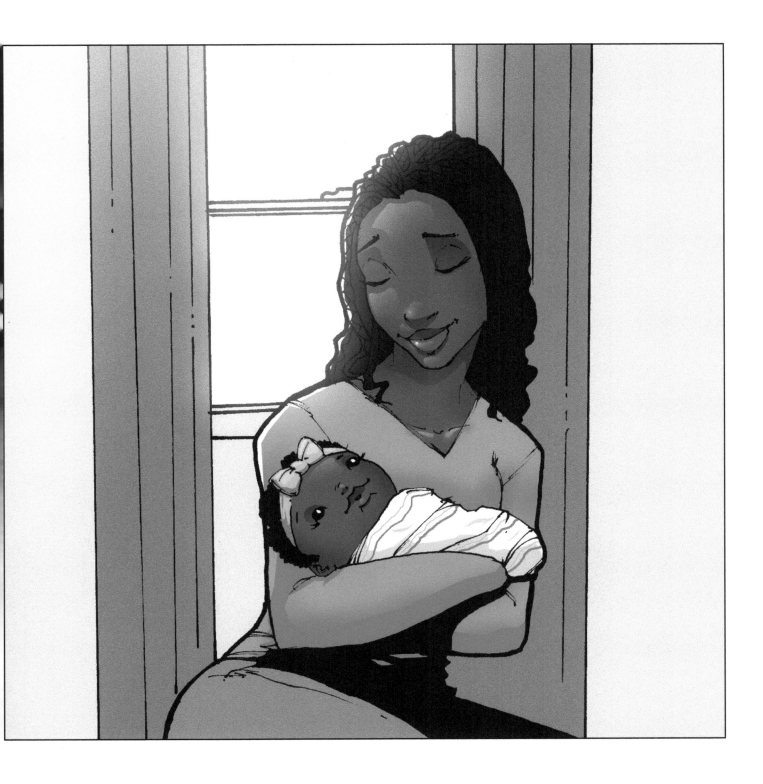

At this time, I did not need any medications or oxygen. The doctors felt that I could wait until I was three to four months before I could have the surgery to repair my heart.

My mother was very, very happy that she finally got to take me home. I needed to be monitored by the cardiologist or heart doctor every week. My mother and grandmother had to monitor me at home for Tet spells. I did not have any episodes while I was at home with them.

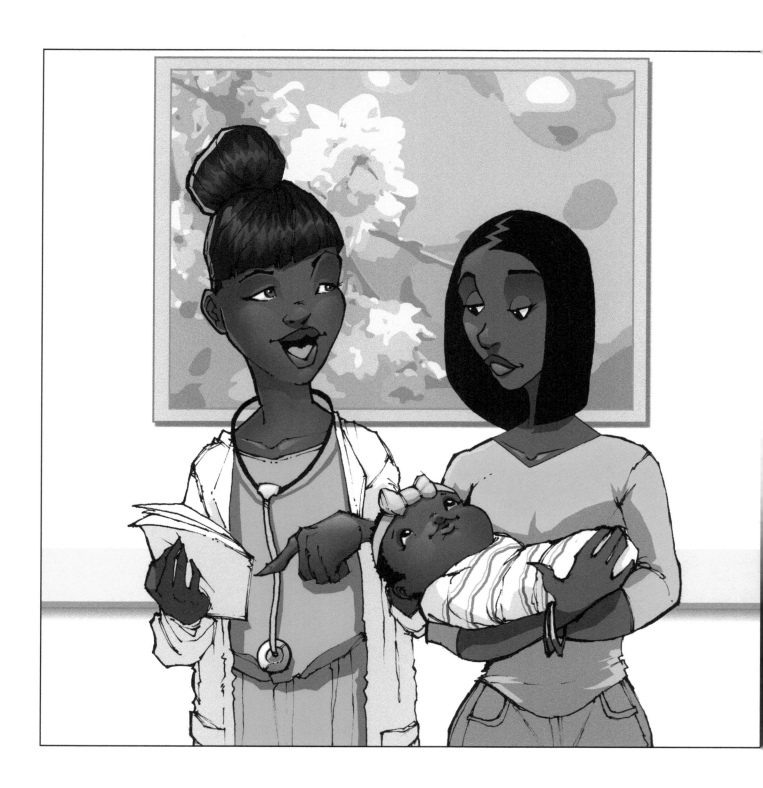

July 12, 2010

I was at home with my mother for 3 weeks. On my second visit to the cardiologist, Doctor Heath had an echocardiogram done. It was discovered that the artery leading to my lungs had narrowed due to the extra tissue. Dr. Heath felt that it would be unsafe for me to go home. I was admitted to the Heart and Kidney Unit again to be monitored until I had heart surgery.

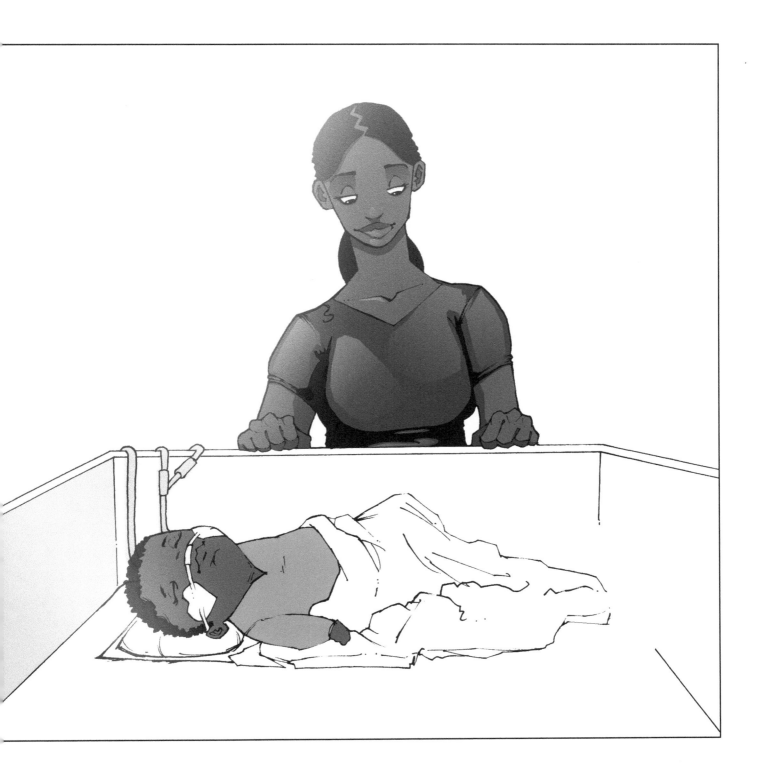

My mother was sad; she began to cry. She wanted me to be home with her. I was placed on oxygen and a medication called Inderal. It was used to decrease my heart rate so that it would not work so hard. I was placed on oxygen because my oxygen levels fell when I started drinking from my bottle or crying.

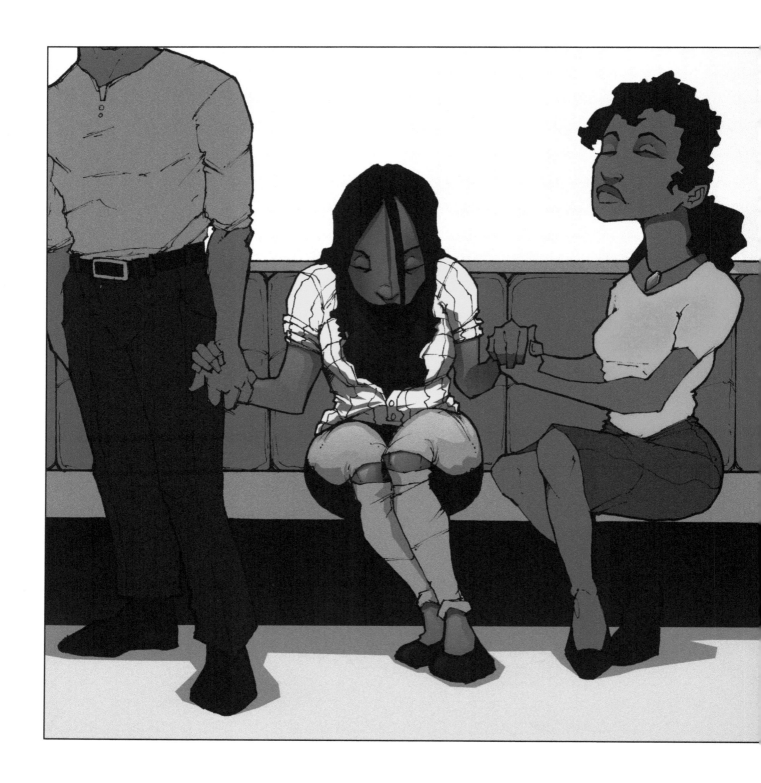

July 21, 2010

After nine days of waiting, the day of my surgery finally arrives. My mother, grandmother, other family members and the members of my church prayed for the nurses, doctors, and I. Doctor Sinha and the surgery team performed my heart surgery. They repaired the hole in my heart and removed the extra tissue so that I could have a new heart. The surgery lasted for four hours, and it was successful. I was taken to the Cardiac Intensive Care Unit after the heart surgery.

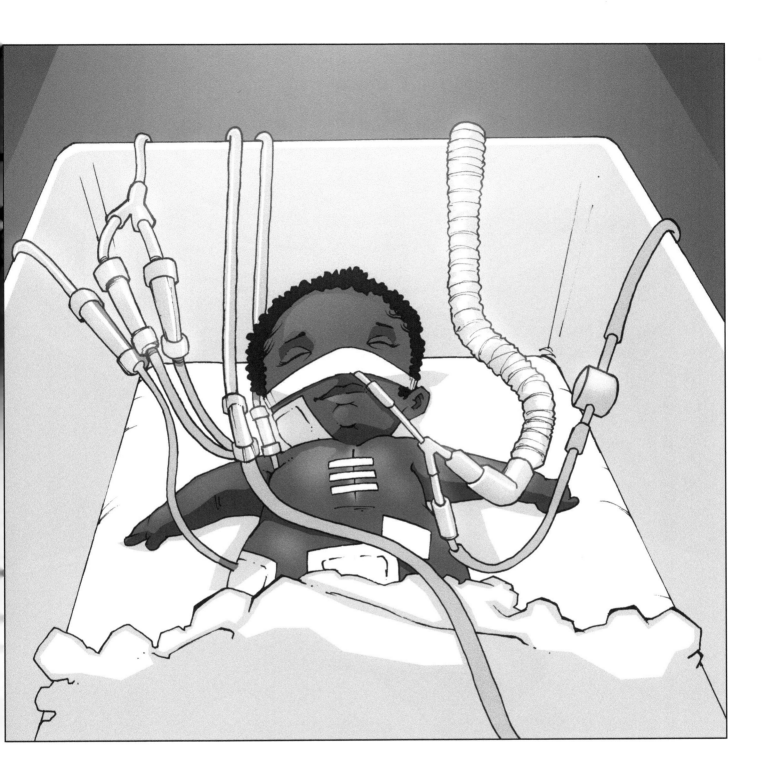

The next few days were rough. Dr. Sinha said my heart was beating too fast. They had to attach a pacemaker to my heart.

I had so many wires and IV tubing attached to me that it scared my mother. Her heart began to hurt, and she cried. For a moment, she lost her faith, but she still continued to pray.

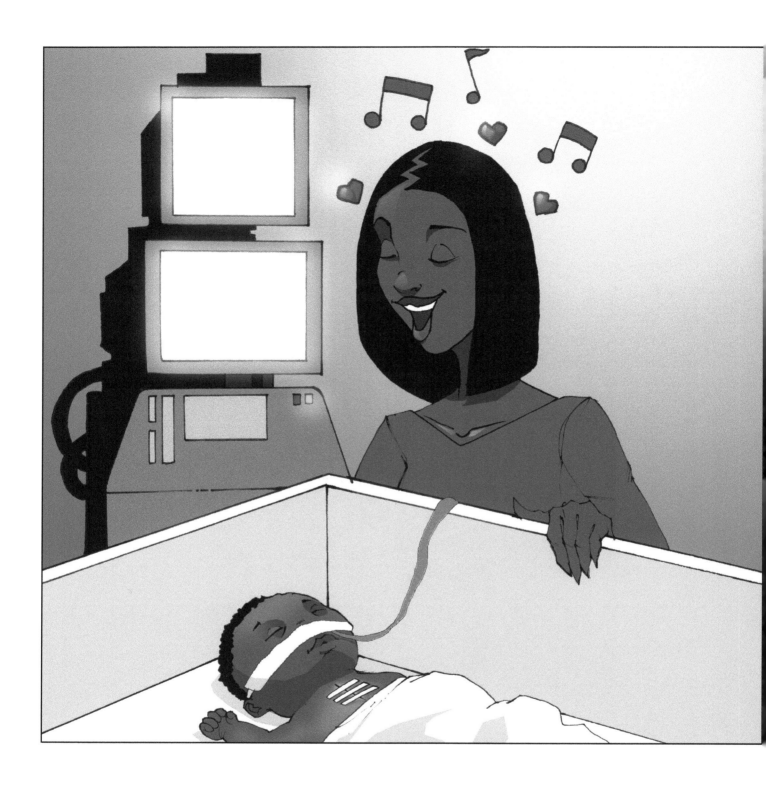

July 23, 2010

I was still on the respirator machine. Each day had some improvement; some tubes were removed. I was sleeping all day because I was given medication to keep me still so that I could continue to heal. My mommy wants to hold me, but she cannot. She continues to touch my hands, talk, and sing to me. I could hear her. I could feel her touch, but I could not respond.

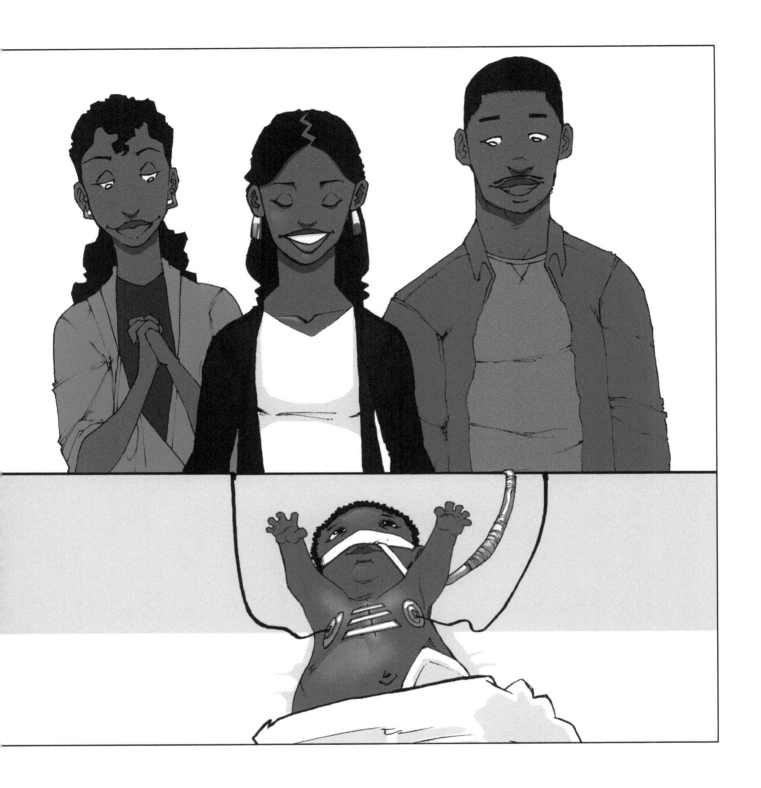

July 24, 2010

Yay! I have been off the pacemaker since 6 AM this morning. My new heart is improving each day. Some of the tubes were removed. Also, I opened my eyes today while mommy, grandma, and grandpa visited.

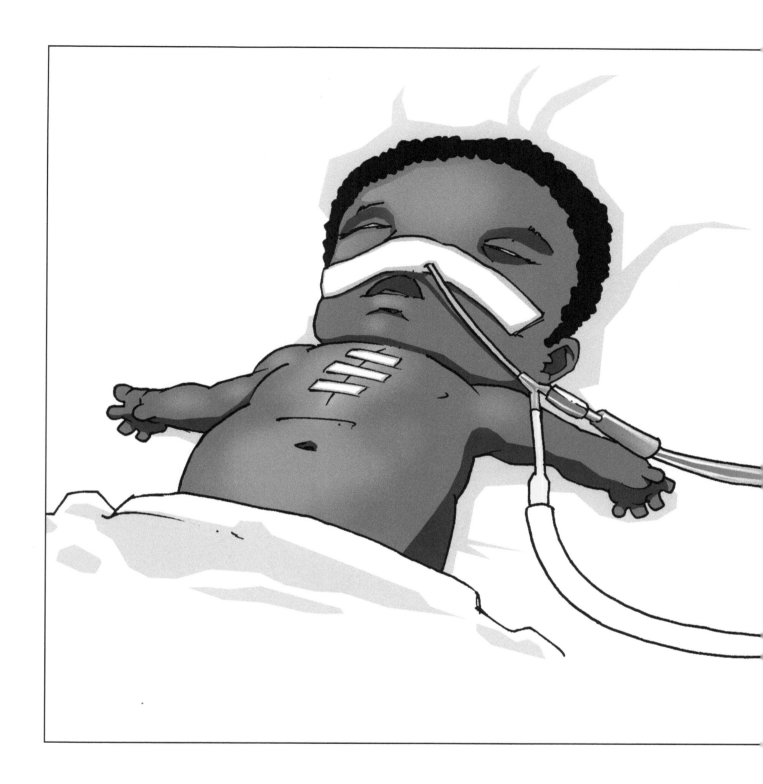

July 25, 2010

The chest tube and the line in my right atrium were removed. I was started on Nasogastric Tube feeding through my nose at a slow rate. If I am able to tolerate it, I would be able to get my bottle.
I CAN'T WAIT!
I am more awake but not completely.

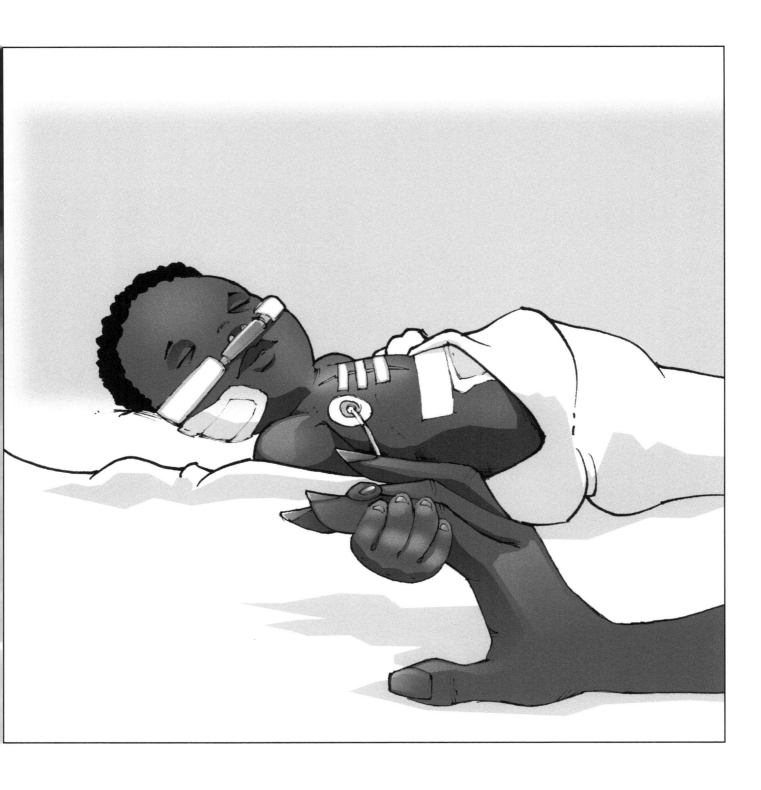

July 26, 2010

I was removed from the respirator which helped me to breathe and the Foley Tube which was used to collect my urine. At first, I had a hard time breathing and had to be given medication to open my breathing tube. I was placed on oxygen through my nose, and by the time my mommy left my side, it was decreased.

I am more awake now. For the first time since July 21st, my mother heard me cry. It was not like my usual cry because I am a little hoarse. At least she heard me cry.   As my mommy sat by my bedside, I looked her in the eyes and held on to her finger for dear life and then I fell asleep.

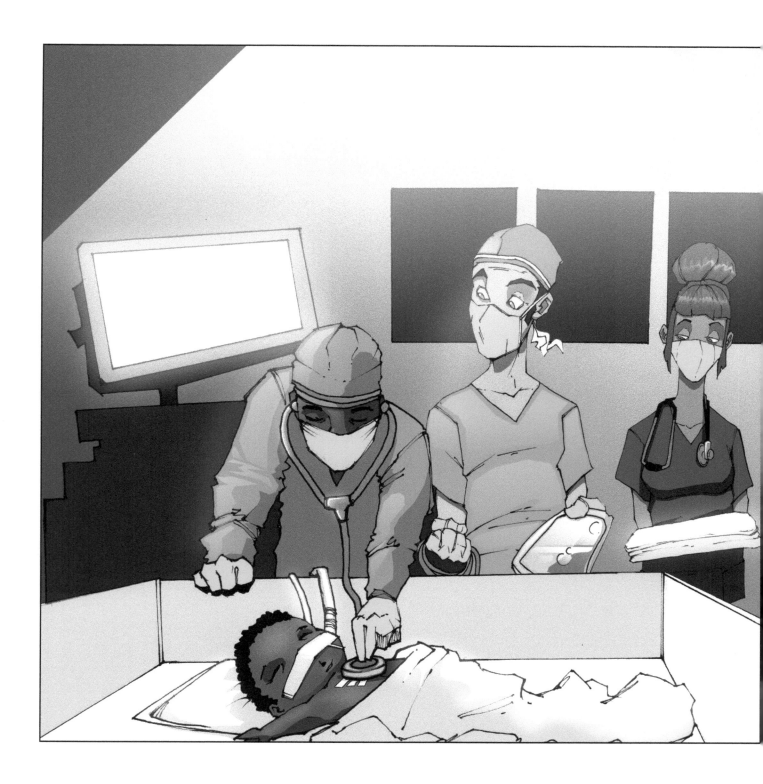

July 27, 2010

I had a rough night last night. I still, have some swelling in my throat. I was placed on a steroid to decrease the swelling. I vomited, so I could not get my bottle. I am still getting my formula through the tube in my nose. Most of the IV fluids have been discontinued, and the IV line I had in my chest was removed. My oxygen was decreased.

Grandpa visited today, and I opened my eyes for him. Dr. Berger, Dr. Spumey and the other doctors and nurses of the Cardiac Unit took good care of me. They got my family and I through this difficult time.

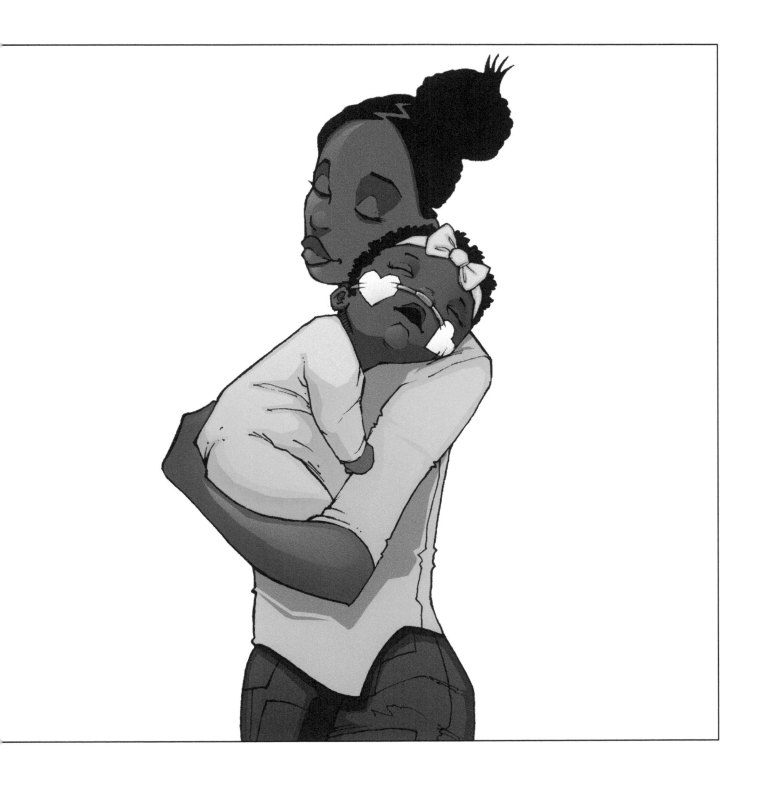

July 28, 2010

Finally, I was taken back to the Heart and Kidney Unit. YAY! YAY! My family and family friends were happy. I am one step closer to going home.

Now, I am on less oxygen. My oxygen levels are excellent. I started to drink my formula out of my bottle, and I tolerated it well. The most important thing about today is that my mother held me in her arms for the first time since July 21st!

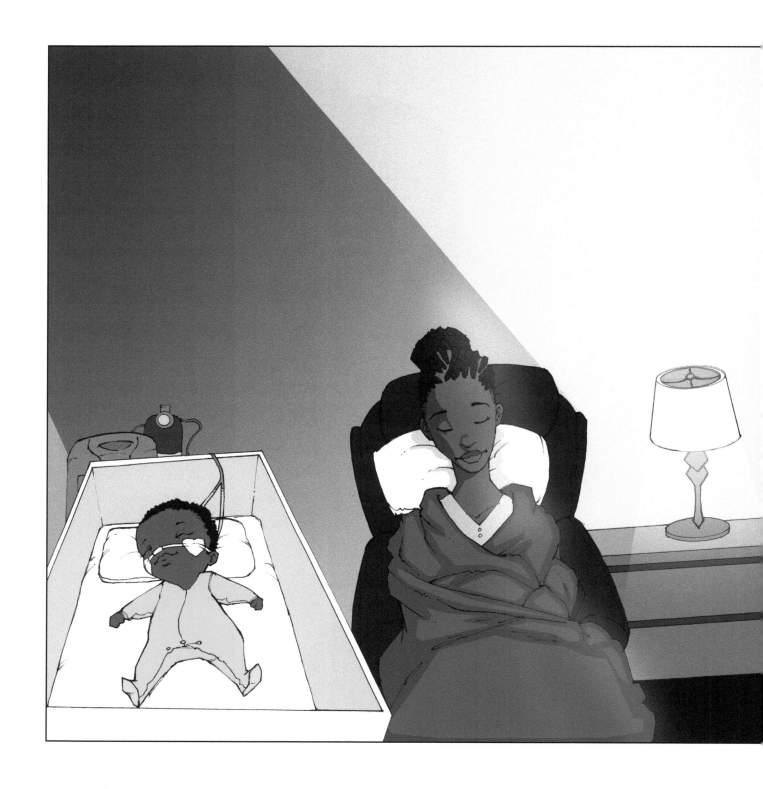

July 29, 2010

I am totally awake. I am on ¼ liter of oxygen. Next step, NO MORE OXYGEN! My mother spent the night with me. I am almost ready to go home. Dr. Beaton said I could go home by the weekend. Mommy and I can't wait to continue bonding at home.

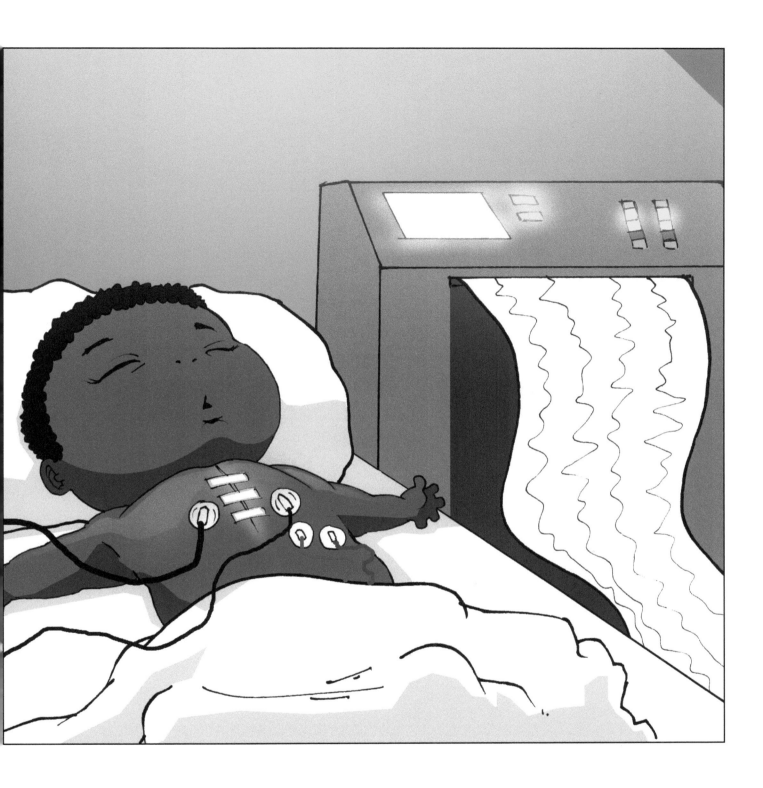

July 30, 2010

My oxygen levels are within normal limits, and my oxygen was discontinued. Finally, they removed the pacemaker connection to my heart. I had an electrocardiogram (EKG) and another echocardiogram done today to make sure my new heart is doing fine. All is well, but my appetite is decreased, and I am sleepy. I have been through a lot for such a little person. I just want to go home.

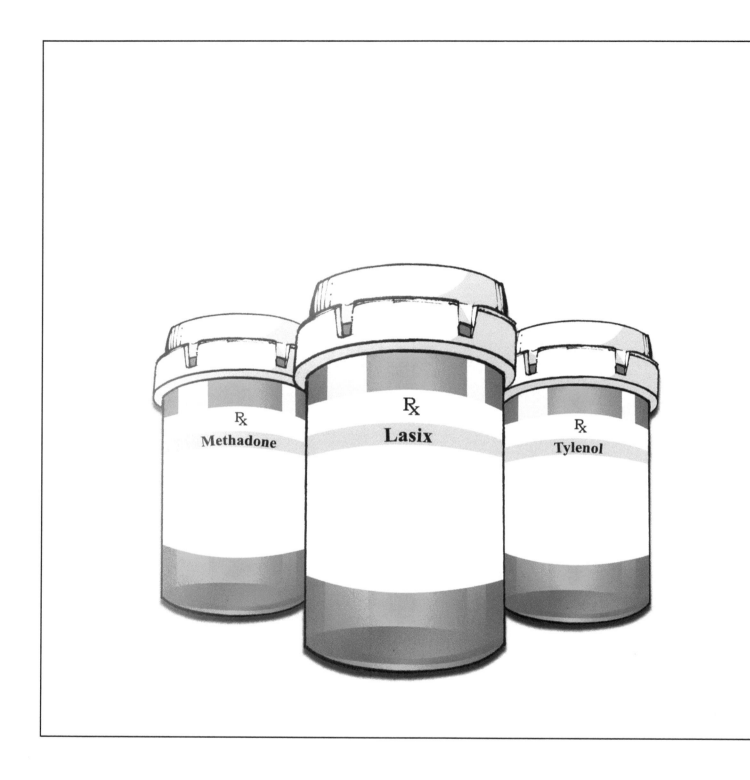

July 31, 2010

1:30 PM – The doctors told my mother that I could go home today. I am so ready to be placed in my stroller and pushed by my mother out the front door of this hospital.

7:30 PM – Finally, I'm going home. I had to wait for one of my medications to be delivered to the hospital.

Home medication: Lasix – To help me get rid of the extra fluids in my body.

Tylenol - For pain and Methadone – to help me wean off the medication they were giving me for pain. I will be weaned off the Methadone by August 16, 2010.

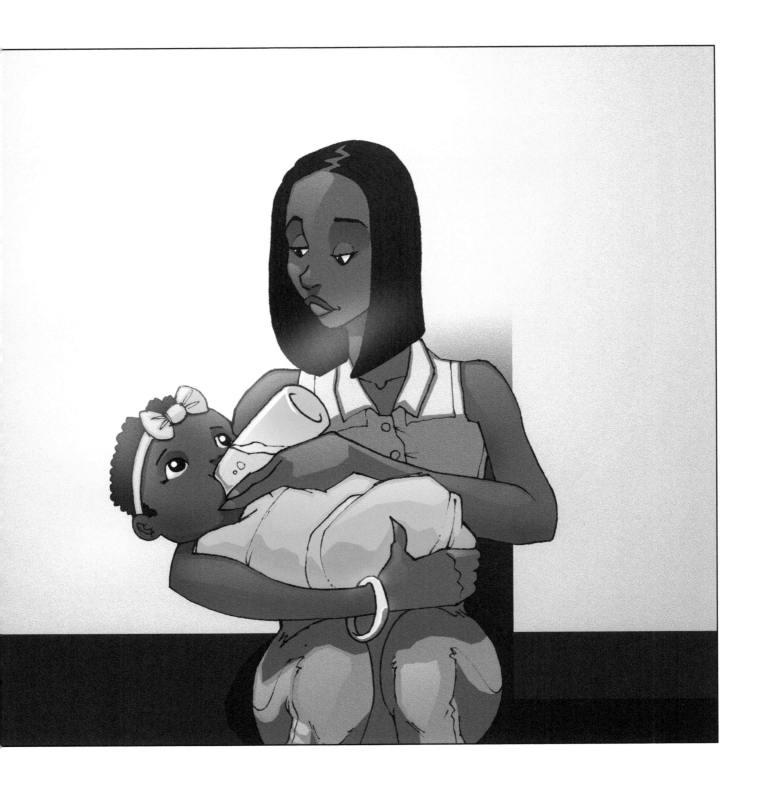

At Home

am doing fine. I get irritable sometimes because of the pain. My incision is healing without any signs of infection. My mother keeps it clean by following the directions given by the doctor and nurse. My appetite is good. I am drinking at least 2 ounces of milk every 2 hours now.

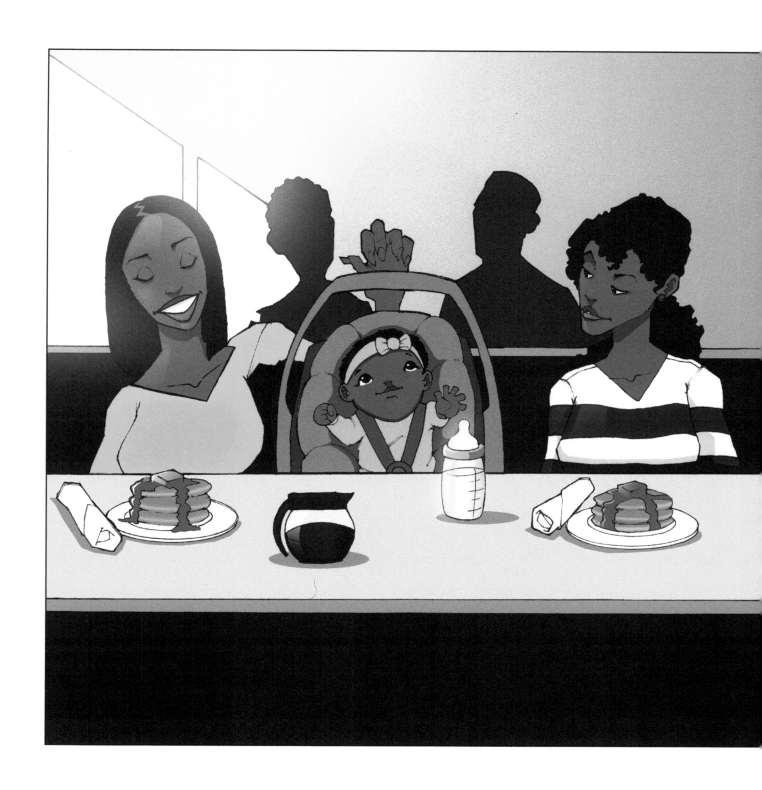

August 7, 2010

First trip out of the house to IHOP. I am celebrating the success of my surgery with mommy and grandma. It has been 2 weeks since my surgery, and it is now safe for me to be around other people. I they want to touch me, they have to wash or sanitize their hands.

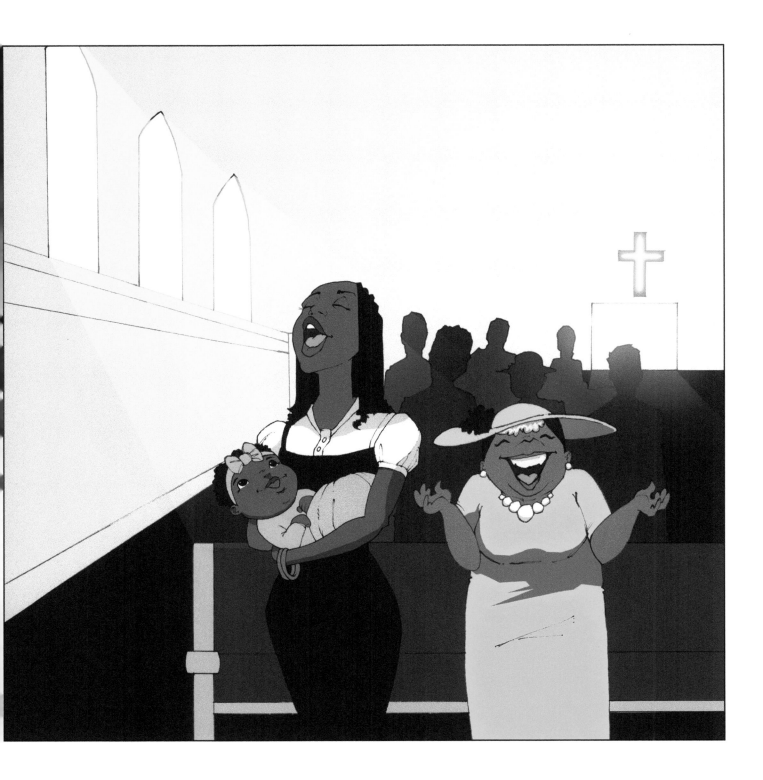

August 8, 2010

I went to church to thank the Lord for all he has done for me.

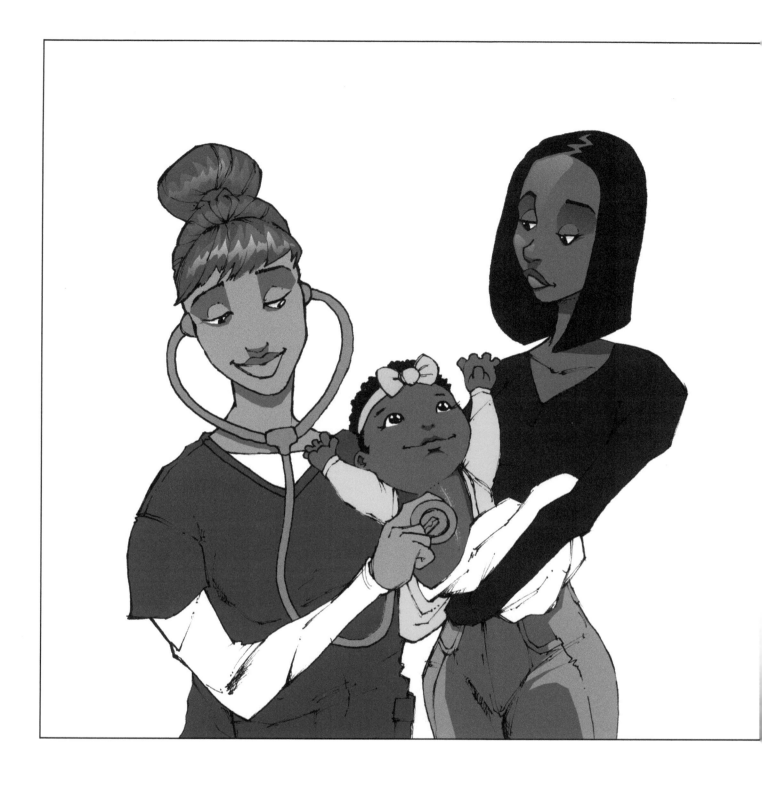

August 10, 2010

I visited Ms. Kathleen Cummins the Cardiovascular Nurse Practitioner at Children's National Medical Center. I had blood work, an electrocardiogram (EKG), and a chest x-ray done. All is well. My oxygen level remained at 95 percent.

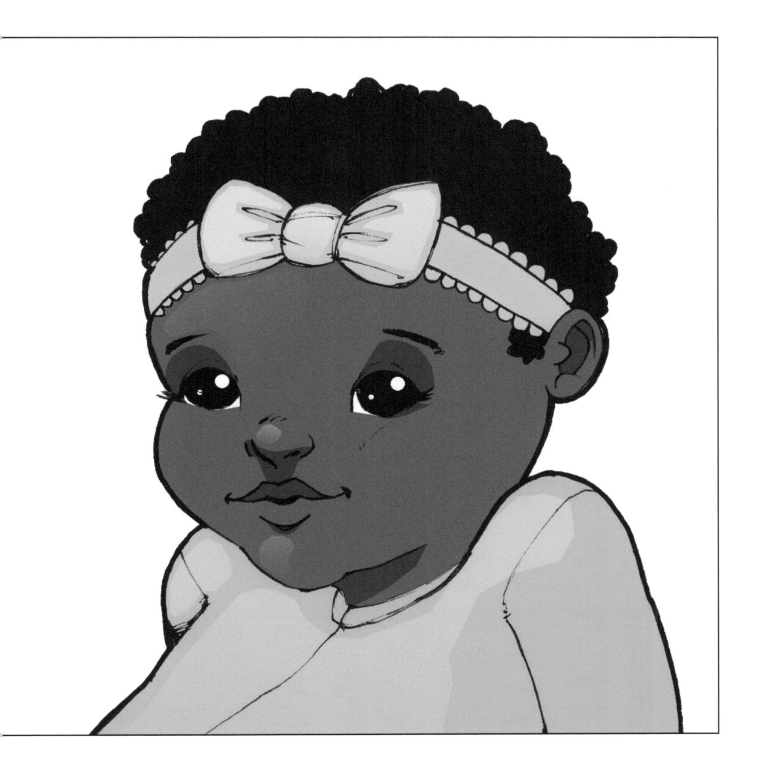

August 16, 2010

I visited Dr. Heath today. An echocardiogram was done, and ALL IS VERY WELL!!! I have been weaned off the Methadone. I no longer need to take the Lasix. I am taking the Tylenol for pain as needed. My incision has healed, and I will return to see Dr. Heath in 2 months. I have come a long way, and by the grace of God, I will continue to be healed.

There's Hope

This was the first of my two open-heart operations. On January 12, 2011, I had a cardiac catheterization. On April 13, 2011, I had my second heart operation. Lastly, I had a stent placed in my heart to widen the artery so my blood could flow better. I need to visit the cardiologist at Children's National Medical Center every year.

Upon genetic testing, it was discovered that my heart condition was related to a genetic disorder called DiGeorge Syndrome, or 22q11.2 deletion. In the 1990's a blood test was developed that identified a missing piece of material on the 22nd chromosome. Children with DiGeorge may have a number of medical and/or educational problems. These can include heart defects, trouble fighting infections, low calcium levels, differences in the roof of the mouth, feeding difficulties, developmental delays, learning disabilities, and behavior problems. However, it is important to remember that most children with DiGeorge do not have problems in every one of these areas. (1)

I have defied the odds. When I was three years old, I enrolled at Jericho Christian Academy. At four years old, I recited the books of the bible. I became a good reader, and I made good grades. I have no problems talking, eating, drinking, walking, or running.

Now, I am 8 years old and about to enter the third grade. I have been reading at the third-grade level. I now attend First Baptist Church of Glenarden, and for Youth Day 2018, I recited the memory verse.

"You are the light of the world. A city that is set on a hill cannot be hidden. Nor do they light a lamp and put it under a basket, but on a lampstand, and it gives light to all who are in the house. Let your light so shine before men, that they may see your good works and glorify your Father in heaven."
Matthew 5: 14-16

"I SHINE"

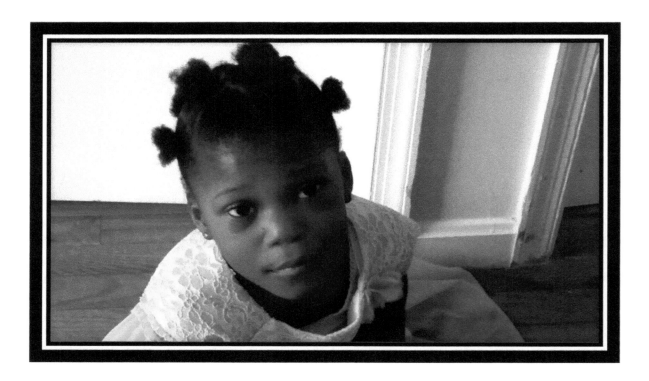

About the Author:

I am Maxine A. Wilson from Kingston, Jamaica. I came to America when I was 11 years old. I graduated from Carlow College in 1984 with a Bachelor of Science Degree in Nursing. I have been a school nurse in Washington, DC since 1999. Currently, I am the school nurse at Ron Brown College Preparatory High School. As far back as I can remember, I have always been interested in expressing myself through writing. I have written short skits, poems, and even a song.

In 2010, when my only child, Judith became pregnant and delivered my granddaughter, Zariah. It was discovered that she had a congenital heart disease. Then, we discovered it was linked to a genetic disorder. It was quite an eye-opener. My heart ached for my daughter and granddaughter.

The Lord placed it upon my heart to begin keeping a journal about what Zariah was experiencing. That journal became "Zariah's New Heart." I want the readers to know that there is always hope. Zariah was not expected to eat, walk or talk on target. She exceeded all expectations. Currently, I live in Maryland with my husband, daughter, and granddaughter, Zariah.